Memory Matters

Healthy and Helpful Recipes that May Prevent Alzheimer's and Dementia

The Health Buff

MP Publishing

Copyright

Table of Contents

Introduction

Packed with delectable dishes, Memory Matters cookbook contains not only easy to prepare but also helpful recipes to avoid brain-harming diseases.

There's no current cure to Alzheimer's and this cookbook will reduce the risk or delay the onset of Alzheimer's and other forms of dementia and memory loss.

The Health Buff is a group of writers that aims to help people on what diet they want to achieve. And this book offers simple and easy mind diet recipes that were gathered in different places.

What is Alzheimer's?

Alzheimer's is a brain disease that forms problems with the affected person's memory, thinking, and behaviors. It is important to emphasize that the memory loss and changes in behavior associated with Alzheimer's are not a normal part of the aging process. Alzheimer's is the most popular form of dementia, a disease for memory loss and other cognitive abilities that is serious enough to interfere with daily life. It is a permanent, progressive brain disorder that will gradually destroys thinking skills and memory and, eventually, the ability to carry out the simplest tasks.

Alzheimer's is not a normal part of aging. The most popular risk factor is increasing age, and the majority of people with Alzheimer's are 65 and older. But this disease is not just a disease of old age.

Alzheimer's disease is named after Dr. Alois Alzheimer in 1906. He observed changes in the brain tissue of a woman who had died with an unusual mental illness.

Currently, there is no cure for Alzheimer's. But drug and non-drug treatments may help with both cognitive and behavioral symptoms.

Researchers are looking for new treatments to modify the course of the disease and improve the quality of life for people with Alzheimer's and dementia.

Causes of Alzheimer's

Age: Everyone's risk for Alzheimer's goes up as they get older. And for most, it starts going up after age 65.

The Family history: People with parent(s) or sibling with Alzheimer's are more likely to get the disease.

Gender: More often than men, women tend to get this disease. This is for one, is because women live longer than men and age are the number one risk factor for Alzheimer's.

Accident/ Head injury: Studies has shown a major link between Alzheimer's disease and accidents/ injuries affecting the head.

Down syndrome: People with this disorder often get Alzheimer's disease at early stages say 30s to 40s.

Other factors include high blood pressure, High cholesterol levels.

Good Food to Prevent Alzheimer's

Green leafy veggies

-       spinach, lettuce, Brussels sprouts, arugula, collard greens, and kale

Variety of non-leafy vegetables

-       squash, beets, tomatoes, peas, endives, zucchini, and eggplant

Nuts

-       almonds, walnuts, cashews, and pistachios

Berries

-       blueberries, raspberries, and strawberries

Whole grains

-       buckwheat, faro, barley, oats, and quinoa

Fish

-       salmon, tuna, trout, and halibut

Poultry Products

-       such as chickens, turkey, geese and duck can be eaten atleast 2 times a week

Olive oil

-       is strongly recommended to use as cooking oil because it consists of healthy fats.

Big Meals for the Healthy Mind

Apricot Glazed Salmon

Here is what you need:

- 1/ 3 cup apricot fruit spread (pure apricot fruit)
- ¼ Tsp black pepper, freshly ground
- 1 Tbsp extra-virgin olive oil
- 1 clove of garlic, minced
- ½ cup vegetable broth (in low sodium)
- 1 Tbsp Dijon mustard
- 1 1⁄3 pounds salmon fillets

Directions:

1. Start by preheating the grill to medium heat.

2. After that, dry the salmon with a paper towel and cut into four equal servings.

3. Now, season the skinless side of salmon with the pepper and place each piece on a double layer of foil with skin side down.

4. And then, fold the sides of the foil up so that the cooking oil will not run out.

5. Beat the rest of the ingredients in a bowl and pour the liquid over the four pieces of salmon so the glaze will spread equally.

6. After which, close each foil by folding as if you were wrapping a gift.

7. When done, slide the foil packets onto the grill and close the lid.

8. Allow to cook until the salmon is cooked through (takes about 10 minutes).

9. When done, let it rest for 2 minutes then unwrap

10. Then serve the salmon!

Salmon Wrapped Asparagus

Here's what you need:

- 10 asparagus spears
- 1 tsp olive oil
- 3 oz. wild caught smoked salmon
- 2 tsp coconut milk
- 1 tsp yellow mustard
- ¼ tsp dried dill

Directions:

1. First, heat the oven to 400F. Then place the asparagus on a foil-lined pan and brush with oil.

2. Roast for 10 minutes, remove from oven and allow to rest on the pan.

3. Prepare the mustard dill sauce by stirring the coconut milk, mix mustard and dill together in a small bowl. When done, wrap slices of smoked salmon around bundles of the asparagus spears (2-3 per bundle).

4. Drizzle with sauce then serve!

Salmon Cakes with Greens

Here's what you need:

- ½ cup fennel, shaved thin
- ½ Tbsp coconut oil
- ¼ cup parsnips (shaved)
- 6 oz can boneless, skinless salmon, dried
- 1 Tbsp quinoa flakes
- 1 Tbsp fresh chives, chopped
- 1 egg
- 1 tsp capers
- 4 radishes & greens
- 1 tsp lemon juice
- 1/ 2 Tbsp coconut oil

Directions:

1. First, heat the oil in a skillet and sauté the fennel and parsnips until tender for about 7 minutes.

2. When done, place on to a serving plate.

3. Proceed by combining the salmon, egg, chives, quinoa flakes, capers, and lemon juice together in a mixing bowl. Mix until most of the large salmon chunks are broken down.

4. After mixing, heat oil in a frying pan on medium heat.

5. Form the salmon mixture into 2 patties and allow cooking for 4 minutes per side.

6. Place salmon cakes over fennel and parsnips and garnish with radishes.

7. Serve warm.

Honey Salmon Steaks and A Sesame Rocket Salad

Here's what you need:

- 4 salmon steaks
- 2 tablespoons of lemon juice
- 3 tablespoons of olive oil
- 3 tablespoons of honey
- 2 tablespoons of sesame seeds
- 1 bag of rocket salad
- 1 lemon, cut into quarters for garnish

Directions:

1. In a frying pan, warm up the olive oil then add the honey and mix well. When the oil is very hot, place the salmon steaks with the skin first to cook.

2. Cook for about 3 to 4 minutes on each side depending on the thickness of the salmon.

3. Meanwhile, put the rocket salad in a large serving bowl.

4. When the salmon steaks are done, remove them from the heat and keep them warm.

5. Add the sesame seeds and cook for about 1 to 2 minutes in the same frying pan.

6. Deglaze immediately with the lemon juice. And after that, pour the dressing onto the rocket salad.

7. Mix well and then season.

8. Serve the salmon either on the top of the rocket salad or on the side.

Healthy Salmon Beet Salad

Here's what you need:

For the salad:

- 170 g salmon flakes, precooked
- 64 g beets, cooked
- 3 cups of romaine lettuce
- 12 pcs. pistachios, chopped
- a quarter of a medium-sized avocado, cut into cubes
- 1 big-sized orange, coarsely chopped
- 1 red onion, finely chopped

For the vinaigrette:

- 2 tbsp. white wine vinegar
- 1 tbsp. olive oil, extra virgin
- ½ tsp. Dijon mustard
- 2 tbsp. orange juice, freshly squeezed
- ½ tsp., orange zest1
- Freshly ground black pepper
- ¼ tsp. chili powder
- a pinch of kosher salt
-

Directions:

1. Mix all of the ingredients for the vinaigrette in a bowl. Beat well until you arrive at a smooth texture.

2. In a salad bowl, combine the salmon and the romaine lettuce.

3. Add the avocado and the orange slices and toss. Add the beets and the onions and toss again.

4. Pour the dressing over the bed of romaine and toss again.

5. Add the pistachio nuts on top before serving.

Fish Filets with Veggies

Here's what you need:

- 4 filets of white fish,
- 1 leeks, finely slice
- 2 carrots, finely slice
- 1 shallot, chopped
- 1 tablespoon of olive oil
- 1 glass of white wine
- 3 tablespoons of single cream
- 1 teaspoon of thyme
- Salt and pepper to taste

Directions:

1. Start by preheating the oven at 350 F.

2. Then heat the olive oil in a frying pan. Add shallot then cook until tender. And following on the shallots, add the leeks and carrots and cook for 5 minutes on low heat.

3. While stirring occasionally, pour the white wine and reduce for another 5 minutes. Add the cream and season. Place the fish fillets first in four small individual oven dishes. Cover with vegetable mixture.

4. Sprinkle the top with thyme. Cook in the oven for about 15 to 20 minutes.

5. Serve hot and enjoy.

Fruity Monkfish Tartar

Here's what you need:

- ½ lb. of monkfish filets
- 8 strawberries
- ¼ watermelon
- 2 avocado
- 1 lemon
- 1 red onion
- 4 tablespoons of olive oil
- 1 tablespoon of vinegar
- 1 teaspoon of honey
- Salt and pepper to taste

Directions:

1. Cut the monkfish into very small cubes then season.

2. Cut the strawberries into small pieces and follow the watermelon into small cubes.

3. Peel and cut the red onion thinly. Cut the avocado into smaller pieces and mix with the lemon juice. Climb the tartar with a kitchen metal circle.

4. First, layer the avocado and layer the fish after. Finish the layering with mix strawberries and watermelon.

5. Mix the olive oil and vinegar in a bowl then add the honey and red onion. Season and then mix well.

6. Pour the dressing on the plate all around the tartar and serve.

Fresh Mussels in Gluten free Beer

Here's what you need:

- 4 tablespoons olive oil
- 1 onion Half leek white part
- Bunch of chives
- Half a celery root
- 15-20 mussels
- 1 cup gluten free beer
- ¼ cup heavy cream
- 1 tablespoon butter
- A Pinch of coarse salt

Directions:

1. Heat a deep pan and add the oil.

2. Slice the onion and leek into thin slices.

3. Heat up the oil in a frying pan; fry the onions and leek until they have softened and golden.

4. Chop the chives, following the celery and parsley.

5. Add the roots then combine and toss everything together.

6. After 2-3 minutes of softening the roots, add the mussels and then toss again.

7. Add the beer, let it all simmer in the pan for a few minutes and reduce the alcohol.

8. Toss occasionally and when the mussels start to open, add the cream and butter.

9. Season with salt lightly, check again if all the mussels opened up and can be moved to a deep serving dish. Sprinkle with chopped chives then serve.

10. Healthy Reminder: Mussels that are open before cooking, and that did not open after cooking is not fresh.

Super Easy Fish Cake

Here's what you need:

- 1.25 kg of fish (Sea bass, Cod or even fresh Salmon), as a whole or fillets
- 6 potatoes – cut into thin round slices
- 3 cloves of garlic – chopped
- Bundle/ bunch of parsley also chopped
- 60 grams of pecorino cheese – grated
- Olive oil
- Salt, pepper, paprika
- Turmeric (optional)

Directions:

1. Oil a medium size baking tray and place half of the potatoes.

2. On the potatoes sprinkle half of the garlic and half of the chopped parsley. Now add the cheese (the whole amount).

3. On top of those ingredients place the fish and season with some pepper, paprika and ¼ teaspoon of turmeric.

4. Now put the rest of the potatoes, parsley and garlic (in that order).

5. Season with pepper, paprika and a little bit of salt and add more olive oil.

6. Place in the oven at 200 Celsius for 30 minutes.

7. Enjoy!

Lamb with Black Olives

Here's what you need:

- 12 oz. boned leg of lamb, cut into cube
- 4 tablespoons of olive oil
- 2 garlic cloves, crushed and chopped
- 1 onion, chopped
- 1 small red chili, deseeded and chopped finely
- ½ cup of white wine
- 6 oz. of stoned black olives
- 1 sprigs of parsley, chopped
- 1 tablespoon of rosemary
- Salt and pepper to taste

Directions:

1. In a frying pan, heat up the olive oil.

2. Put the onion, garlic and red chili onto the pan then cook until tender.

3. Add the lamb and brown from all sides and be sure not to burn it.

4. Deglaze with the white wine for 2 to 3 minutes.

5. Add the black olive and lower the heat to medium.

6. Add the rosemary and season.

7. Then cook and simmer for 20 minutes.

8. Stir occasionally during the last 5 minutes, add half of the parsley.

9. Transfer the lamb into a serving dish.

10. Sprinkle some parsley then serve and enjoy.

Minted Pesto Lamb Salad

Here's what you need:

- 1.5 lb. lamb, cooked and sliced
- 1 onion, sliced
- 2 garlic cloves, crushed
- 1 salad of your choice
- 1 red pepper, cut into strips
- 1 yellow pepper, cut into strips
- 2 tablespoons of pine nuts
- 2 oz. of fresh basil
- 1 oz. of fresh mints
- ½ cup of olive oil
- Salt and pepper to taste

Directions:

1. Prepare the salad in a large bowl.

2. Add red and yellow peppers then the onion and mix well.

3. Put the pine nuts, basil, and mints in a blender then season. Start blending and add the olive oil little by little until you get to a smooth paste.

4. Put four portions of salad on four plates. Add the slice of lamb on the top.

5. Drizzle some of the minted pesto on each plate.

6. Serve and enjoy.

Mushroom Chicken

Here's what you need:

- 2 onions cut into rings
- ¼ cup oil
- 15 fresh mushrooms sliced
- 600 gram of clean chicken breast cut into long strips
- 3 teaspoons gluten free mushroom soup powder
- 1 cup water

Directions:

1. In a preheated and oiled deep pan, fry the onions until softened.

2. Add the chicken and fry on each side for about 2-3 minutes and put aside.

3. Add the mushrooms to the onions and cook for 5 minutes.

4. Add mushroom soup powder and water.

5. Put the chicken back in the pan and cook in a low heat for 15 minutes.

6. Serve in your best serving dish and enjoy.

Chicken Mediterranean Casserole

Here's what you need:

- 1 whole chicken cut into 8 pieces
- 1 onion, chopped
- 2 garlic cloves, crushed
- 1 zucchini, sliced
- 1 yellow bell pepper, cut into strips
- 1 red bell pepper, cut into strips
- 6 oz. of button mushrooms, sliced
- 6 tomatoes, sliced
- 1 Tablespoon of thyme
- 1 bay leaf 4 oz. of green olives, stoned
- ½ cut of red wine
- ½ cup of chicken stock
- 2 tablespoons of olive oil
- Salt and pepper to taste

Directions:

1. Start by preheating the oven at 350 F. Warm up the olive oil in a large sauce pan. Fry the chicken pieces on each side until they have a nice golden brown color.

2. Remove the chicken and place in the oven dish. Add and sweat the onion and garlic until tender. Put the onion and garlic into the oven dish.

3. Add the red and yellow peppers, and zucchini.

4. Add the mushrooms, tomatoes, and the green olives.

5. Add the thyme and bay leaf then season. Pour the red wine and the chicken stock. Cook and simmer in the oven for about 45 minutes. Remove from the oven and make sure the chicken is thoroughly cooked.

6. Serve while hot.

Grilled Chicken with Endives and Cashew and Raisins Salad

Here's what you need:

- 2 endives, shredded
- ½ cos lettuce, shredded
- 4 chicken breasts
- 2 tablespoons of olive oil
- 1 red onion, sliced
- 1 cup of unsalted cashew
- 1 cup of dry raisins
- 1 cup of yogurt
- 2 garlic cloves, finely chopped
- ¼ cup of lemon juice
- ¼ cup of coriander, chopped
- Salt and pepper to taste

Directions:

1. Flatten the chicken breasts with a kitchen hammer or with your rolling pin. Brush the chicken with the olive oil. Cook the flattened chicken under the grill until it is done.

2. Combine the yogurt with the garlic, lemon juice, and coriander in a bowl.

3. Mix well and leave on the side. Combine the endives with the cos lettuce in a large serving bowl.

4. Add the red onion, cashew and raisins. Mix everything well.

5. Toss gently then slowly, the yogurt dressing will combine with the salad. Slice the grilled chicken and place it on the top of the salad.

6. Serve and enjoy.

Thai Style Chicken Salad Wraps

Here's what you need:

- ¼ cup mayonnaise
- 2 tablespoons fresh grated ginger
- 2 tablespoons honey
- 2 tablespoons fresh lime juice
- 2 tablespoons plain yogurt
- 1 teaspoon Thai red curry paste
- 1 ½ cups cooked chicken, diced or shredded in a food processor
- ½ cup pineapple tidbits, drained
- ¼ cup chopped fresh cilantro
- ¼ cup slivered almonds
- 4 gluten-free tortilla wraps
- 1 cup baby spinach, washed and spun dry

Directions:

1. First, in a medium bowl, stir together the mayonnaise, ginger, honey, lime juice, yogurt, curry paste, chicken, pineapple, cilantro, and almonds, until blended altogether.

2. Soften the tortilla wraps and immediately lay the tortillas on wax paper on a flat surface.

3. Spread ¼ of the chicken salad over a tortilla. Top with ¼ cup spinach.

4. Then gently roll tortilla into a loose roll, and then cut in half diagonally.

5. Repeat the process with the remaining tortillas, filling, and spinach.

6. Serve immediately.

Veggie Pie

Here's what you need:

- 4 medium sized potatoes
- 4 zucchini
- 4 carrots
- ¾ cup oil 1 tablespoon of gluten free chicken soup powder
- Parsley and Dill
- 1 ½ cups gluten-free flour
- ½ pack baking powder
- Salt and pepper to taste

Directions:

1. Peel the potatoes, carrots and zucchini then grate them coarsely.

2. Place in a large bowl, add all the other ingredients and mix well.

3. In a baking tray covered with a baking sheet, place all the ingredients together and flatten.

4. Bake for 1 hour on a medium heat of 180 C or 360 F.

5. Remove immediately on the oven then serve.

Eggplant Lasagna

Here's what you need:

- 2 large eggplants (sliced ¼" thick lengthwise)
- 1 med yellow onion, chopped
- 2 cloves garlic, minced
- 1 pkg (14– 16 oz) firm tofu, drained
- 1 Tbsp olive oil
- 1 jar (24 oz.) marinara sauce
- 6 oz shredded dairy-free mozzarella-style cheese
- 10 oz cremini mushrooms (sliced)
- ½ cup chopped fresh parsley
- 1 Tbsp freshly grated lemon zest

Directions:

1. First, place tofu in a fine mesh strainer over a bowl and set aside.

2. After that, heat the oven to 375 ° F. Coat the eggplant with cooking spray and arrange on 2 sheet pans lightly coated with cooking spray.

3. Roast until lightly browned, it will take about 12 minutes.

4. When done, heat oil in a large skillet over medium heat and add the onion and garlic and cook for 5 to 6 minutes or until soft.

5. Include the mushrooms and cook until tender for 8 minutes before adding the marinara sauce, reserving ½ cup, and bring to a boil.

6. Allow to simmer for a few minutes until slightly thickened. 8. Put the tofu in a medium sized bowl with lemon zest, parsley, and half of the cheese.

7. Stir for a while and spread remaining ½ cup marinara sauce evenly in a 13 by 9" baking pan. Layer one-third of the eggplant the pan and top with one-third of the tofu/ lemon zest mixture and one-third of the marinara sauce: repeat this twice.

8. Finally, sprinkle with the remaining cheese and bake for 25 minutes or until eggplant tender.

9. Allow to cool for 20 minutes then cut. Serve and enjoy.

Mushroom and Spinach with Poached Egg

Here's what you need:

- 1 medium mushroom, any kind you like
- 1/ 16 teaspoon garlic salt
- ½ tablespoon butter
- 1 cup fresh baby spinach, measured by pressing into cup
- 1 tomato slice
- 1 poached egg
- A sprinkle of Parmesan cheese
- salt and pepper, to taste

Directions:

1. Wash mushroom and slice into microwave-safe cup then add garlic salt and butter.

2. Then microwave on high settings for 1 minute.

3. Spread onto serving plate.

4. Wash spinach and place in microwave-safe cup. Spinach should be damp.

5. After washing, microwave spinach on high settings for at least 45 seconds. Drain excess water. Pile spinach on top of the mushrooms.

6. Place tomato slice on top of spinach. Poach egg and place on top of tomato.

7. Sprinkle Parmesan cheese, salt, and pepper on top.

8. Serve immediately and enjoy.

Roasted Chicken with Herbs

Here's what you need:

- 1.3 kg chicken drumsticks, organic (with the skin on)
- 1 tbsp. olive oil
- 1 tsp. thyme
- 11 pcs fresh sage

Directions:

1. Wash and dry the sage. Gently, lift the skin away from the flesh of the chicken and fill each drumstick with equal amounts of dried sage leaves. Make sure that the herb covers about one half of the meat.

2. Heat up the oven to 375 F. And then, spread olive oil at the bottom of a glass baking pan. Roll the marinated drumsticks in the pan so that each piece is totally coated with oil.

3. Arrange the chicken drumsticks in the baking dish with the skin side down. Use half a teaspoonful of the thyme to sprinkle on top of the chicken meat. Place the glass dish in the oven and bake for about 26-43 minutes.

4. After that, flip the meat over. Sprinkle with the remaining half a teaspoonful of thyme. Continue baking for another 19-21 minutes.

5. When the skin is crispy, it should show a nice golden color. Now, serve the dish with some potatoes or rice on other veggies for options.

Veggie Salad Roast

Here's what you need:

- 1 cup eggplant (cubed)
- ½ Tbsp olive oil
- 1 cup shredded cabbage
- 1 Tbsp hemp hearts (hulled hemp seeds)
- 2 tsps sesame seeds
- 4 Kalamata olives
- ½ cup butternut squash (cubed)
- 1 cup dark leafy greens
- 1 hard-boiled egg (sliced)
- Salt and pepper to taste
- Paprika (optional for garnish)

Directions:

1. First, preheat your oven to 425 F and line a baking sheet with foil.

2. Next, toss the eggplant and butternut squash cubes with the olive oil and place on pan.

3. Roast for about 25 minutes, or until they reach desired tenderness.

4. Meanwhile, place the cabbage and greens in a salad bowl. Top with the sesame seeds and hemp hearts followed by the sliced egg.

5. When done roasting the vegetables, arrange them along the
    sides of the salad.

6. Add olives, paprika, salt and pepper to taste.

Broccoli with Balsamic Mushrooms

Here's what you need:

- 1 pound broccoli, cut into 1-inch florets, with stems peeled if desired
- 3 tbsps extra-virgin olive oil, divided
- 8 oz. shiitake mushrooms (stems removed, and caps sliced ½ inch thick)
- 4 oz. baby Bella mushrooms, quartered
- ¼ tsp salt
- 2 large cloves garlic, minced
- 1 tbsp butter
- 2 tbsps balsamic vinegar
- 1 tbsp reduced-sodium tamari
- ¼ tsp crushed red pepper

Directions:

1. First, cook the broccoli in a pot of boiling water until become tender for 3-14 minutes.

2. After that, drain and heat 2 tbsps of oil in a large skillet over medium-high heat.

3. Add the shiitakes and baby bellas then sprinkle with the ¼ tsp salt and cook, stirring often, until deep brown in spots that will take 5 – 8 minutes.

4. When done, reduce heat to medium. Add the garlic along with the remaining 1 tbsp oil and cook, stirring, for 30 seconds.

5. Include the vinegar and tamari, and cook for 30 seconds more. After which you remove from heat and stir in butter, broccoli, and crushed red pepper then gently toss to combine.

6. Serve and enjoy.

Easy Cilantro Pesto

Here's what you need:

- 2 cups spiral cut zucchini (zucchini "noodles")
- ½ cup packed fresh cilantro
- 2 Tbsps olive oil
- 1 Tbsp chopped raw almonds
- ½ tsp minced garlic
- Salt and pepper, to taste

Directions:

1. First, make the zucchini noodles using a spiral vegetable cutting tool.

2. After that, place in a serving bowl and set aside.

3. Blend the cilantro, olive oil, almonds and garlic in a blender until smooth.

4. Toss pesto with the zucchini noodles.

5. Add salt and pepper as needed.

6. Serve and enjoy.

Vegetables in Olive Oil

Here's what you need:

- 2 carrots
- 1 yellow pepper
- 2 small zucchini
- 1 eggplant 1 onion (yellow or red)
- 3 celery sticks
- 1 red pepper
- 1 orange pepper
- ¼ cup of tomato juice
- 2 cloves of garlic
- 12 green olives – chopped
- Olive oil
- 2 tablespoons of fresh thyme, if dry – use a little
- 1 teaspoon of salt 1 teaspoon of pepper, to taste

Directions:

1. Chop the vegetable into cubes.

2. In a large and deep pan heat some olive oil and add the garlic. Fry it till it's browned and take it out. Add the onion and cook for 3-4 minutes.

3. Add the carrots and celery sticks and mix well. Cook for 10 minutes and stir.

4. Add the eggplant and mix well, add the rest of the vegetables and mix well.

5. Add the tomato juice and season and mix everything well. When everything is bubbling, lower the heat and cook half covered for atleast 30 minutes. Add the olives in the last 10 minutes of the cooking process.

6. Serve warm and enjoy.

Turkey and Kale Soup

Here's what you need:

- 250 g turkey
- 40 oz. chicken stock, organic
- 32 oz. kale 3 medium-sized carrots, shaved
- 12 oz. cauliflower, minced
- 15 oz. fresh tomatoes
- 2 tbsp. olive oil
- 4 shallots
- 1 bell pepper
- Sea salt and black pepper, to taste

Directions:

1. Chop the shallots. Dice the carrots and slice the bell pepper. Cut in the tomatoes into chunks. Remove the ribs from the kale and chop up the leaves.

2. Adjust the stove's setting into medium high. In a saucepan, add the olive oil then heat it up. After that, throw in the chopped shallots, cauliflowers, carrots, and bell pepper.

3. Sauté the veggies for about 9 minutes or until they are almost tender. Next, add the turkey meat and cook for approximately 7 – 10 minutes. Pour in the chicken broth; then followed by the tomatoes. Sprinkle desired amount of salt and pepper.

4. Allow the soup to boil. When it starts to boil, add the kale. Adjust the stove's setting to low and tend to the soup with continuous stirring. Afterwards, replace the lid of the saucepan and leave to simmer for about 13-16 minutes.

5. Serve hot and enjoy.

Vegetable Soup with Barley

Here's what you need:

- 32 g. dry barley
- 32 oz. water
- 1 tbsp. olive oil
- 2 oz. carrots, diced
- ½ tsp. garlic, finely chopped
- 2 oz. onions, yellow variety, diced
- 9 oz. button mushrooms, sliced
- 2 oz. green peas
- 2 tbsp. tamari sauce, low-sodium
- 2 oz. potatoes, diced
- 1 tsp. sea salt and black pepper, to taste

Directions:

1. After rinsing the barley, place it in a big saucepan and pour in the water. Then, leave it to boil. Once the water boils, adjust the stove's setting to low. Replace the lid of the saucepan and allow it to simmer for about 22 minutes.

2. Add the low-sodium tamari. Stir well. Get a smaller pan and adjust the stove's setting to medium heat. Add the olive oil and sauté the garlic and the onions until the latter is soft. Throw in the mushrooms and sauté until tender.

3. Then, transfer the sautéed ingredients into the bigger saucepan with the soup. Next, add the potatoes and the carrots into the broth.

4. Replace the lid of the saucepan and simmer for about 23 minutes. The potatoes should be soft by then. Finally, turn off the heat and add the peas.

5. Season with salt and paper for better tasting then serve.

Creamy Coconut Milk and Chicken Soup

Here's what you need:

- 3 – 4 oz boneless skinless chicken breast (cut into cubes)
- 1 tsp organic unrefined coconut oil
- 1 tsp pure sesame oil
- 1 green onion (thinly sliced)
- 1 tsp fresh garlic (minced)
- 1 small cucumber (thinly sliced)
- ½ tsp curry powder (mild or hot)
- 1 cup low sodium all-natural chicken stock
- ¼ cup pure coconut milk (full fat)
- 2 fresh basil leaves
- Lime wedge and fresh cilantro, for garnish

Directions:

1. First, toss the chicken with sesame oil and cook-stir in a saucepan over high heat until almost cooked through.

2. When done, set the heat to medium and add the coconut oil, garlic, green onion, and curry powder.

3. Cook-stir for 2 minutes and pour in the stock and coconut milk. After that, increase the heat to bring to a boil.

4. Once that is achieved, reduce heat and cover to simmer for at least 15 minutes.

5. When done, pour soup into a serving bowl.

6. Finally, add cucumber, basil and a squeeze of lime then serve!

Tasty Pumpkin Patties

Here's what you need:

- 15 oz. pureed pumpkin
- 15 oz. kidney beans
- 1 tsp. capers, chopped
- 1 big egg, organic
- 2 tbsp. spring onions, chopped
- 50 g breadcrumbs
- 1 tbsp. cilantro
- 1 tbsp. olive oil
- 2 tsp. lime juice
- 68 g flour
- sea salt and black pepper, to taste

Directions:

1. Pour the pumpkin puree into a food processor. Throw in the beans and the capers as well.

2. Add the spring onion, the lime juice, and the cilantro. Add half a teaspoonful of sea salt. Process until completely mixed.

3. Next, break the egg and add it into the mixture. This is to be followed by the breadcrumbs. Mix well, making sure that you spread the egg and the crumbs evenly. Add salt and black pepper for seasoning.

4. Afterwards, create patties by shaping the mixture into even-sized balls and flattening them with your palms. Sprinkle flour over a clean, flat work area. Slap each side of each patty on the flour so both sides are covered. Adjust the stove's setting to medium-high. Heat the olive oil in a big pan. Cook the patties.

5. Three minutes on each side should suffice. You'll know they're ready when they yield a nice golden brown color.

Healthy, Easy Mini Meals and Snacks

Healthy Veggie Pizza Wraps

Here's what you need:

- 4 gluten-free tortilla wraps
- 1 cup store-bought pizza sauce
- 1 cup grated mozzarella cheese
- 1 cup chopped marinated artichokes, drained
- 1 cup baby spinach, rinsed and spun dry
- 4 roasted red peppers, sliced into thin vertical strips
- ¼ cup grated Parmesan cheese

Directions:

1. First, soften the tortillas and immediately lay the tortilla on wax paper on a flat surface.

2. Spread ¼ cup pizza sauce over each tortilla. Top each tortilla with ¼ cup each mozzarella cheese, artichokes, and spinach. Add roasted red pepper strips to each tortilla.

3. Sprinkle each tortilla with 1 tablespoon Parmesan cheese. Carefully roll one of each tortilla into a loose wrap and

wrap it in wax paper, twisting the ends of the wax paper to hold the wrap in place.

4. Place the tortilla wraps in a microwave oven and heat on low 1 to 3 minutes until the cheese is warm or starts to melt. Remove from the micro- wave and slice the wraps in half diagonally.

5. Serve immediately.

Easy Healthy Tuna Pie

Here's what you need:

- 2 cans of tuna – drained
- 3 eggs
- ½ can of corn
- ¼ cup of chopped green olives
- 2 cooked and mashed potatoes
- 8 chopped mushrooms fresh
- Salt, pepper and cumin
- For topping: 1 beaten egg and sesame seeds

Directions:

1. Mix all the ingredients together.

2. Place everything in a square baking pan and bake for 20 minutes on a medium heat - 180 Celsius or 360 Fahrenheit.

3. After 20 minutes in the oven, remove the pan and spread beaten egg and sprinkle the sesame seeds on top.

4. Bake for an additional 20 minutes.

5. Serve and enjoy.

Tuna and Avocado in Green Leafy Wraps

Here's what you need:

- 1 can tuna
- 2 tbsp mayo
- 2 tbsp diced green chiles
- ½ very ripe avocado
- ¼ cup green olives
- 2 large leaves of green leaf lettuce
- 1 scallion

Directions:

1. Simply cut the olives in half and dice scallion.

2. Mash the avocado until creamy and mix together with the mayo.

3. Now combine everything together excluding the lettuce leaf and mix well.

4. Finally, place 1 scoop of tuna salad on each lettuce leaf and enjoy!

Toasted Chickpeas

Here's what you need:

- 16 oz. chickpeas, cooked
- 1 tsp. ground cumin
- 1 tsp. chili powder
- 1 tbsp. olive oil
- ¼ tsp. paprika
- sea salt
- black pepper

Directions:

1. Heat up the oven to 400 F. Before roasting the chickpeas, toss them in the olive oil. Coat them with the chili, then with the cumin, and then with the paprika.

2. Arrange the chickpeas evenly into a baking pan lined with parchment. Sprinkle with desired amount of pepper and just a little bit of natural sea salt. Roasting time is between 33 to 37 minutes.

3. The chickpeas should be crispy and they should yield a beautiful golden brown hue. Be sure to stir the peas from time to time so they won't end up sticking.

4. Serve alone as a snack or for breakfast.

5. Healthy Note: Keep in airtight container to last for 7 days.

Tuna Patties with a Touch of Asian Barbecue Sauce

Here's what you need:

For the patties:

- 3 cans (6 ounces each) canned tuna, drained
- ½ cup gluten-free bread crumbs
- 1 large egg
- 1 tablespoon wheat-free tamari soy sauce
- 1 tablespoon Dijon mustard
- 1 teaspoon chopped fresh thyme, or ½ teaspoon dried
- ½ teaspoon salt
- ½ teaspoons freshly ground black pepper
- 8 pineapple slices
- Paprika, for garnish

For the sauce:

- 1/3 cup gluten-free hoisin sauce
- ¼ cup canola oil
- 1 tablespoon sesame oil
- 1 tablespoon honey
- 1 tablespoon gluten-free Worcestershire sauce
- 1 teaspoon ground ginger
- 1 garlic clove, minced
- 1/8 teaspoon ground cayenne

Directions:

For the sauce:

1. In a small bowl, whisk together the Asian Barbecue Sauce ingredients. Refrigerate up to 1 day. 2

For the burgers:

2. In a medium bowl, combine the tuna, bread crumbs, egg, soy sauce, mustard, thyme, salt, and pepper until well blended. Make 4 patties.

3. In a large non-stick pan or skillet— or on a grill— cook the burgers until done, turning to brown the burgers on both sides, about 4 to 6 minutes per side.

4. Garnish with dash of paprika.

5. Serve with sauce and pineapple slices. Enjoy!

Dried Fruit, Nuts and Feta Salad

Here's what you need:

- ½ cup olive oil
- 3 cloves garlic smashed
- 3 branches of thyme
- Whole cup mixed nuts (Your Favorite Kind)
- Cup of chopped dried fruit (they like)
- Chili Coarse salt Black pepper
- ¼ cup white wine
- 1 package washed spinach leaves
- ½ cup fresh basil leaves
- Two separate branches of mint leaves
- Pinch of chili pepper or 100g sheep feta
- 1 tablespoon Silan

Directions:

1. Heat half the olive oil in large skillet over medium heat. Sauté garlic and thyme, stirring constantly for about 3 minutes.

2. Add the nut mixture and fry for about 7 minutes on low heat. Turn up the flame and add the dried fruit mixture.

3. Season with chili, salt and pepper for better tasting. Stir for a minute and add the wine. Cook for 2 minutes and remove from heat.

4. On a large serving dish sprinkle the spinach leaves, basil and mint. Sprinkle the stew over them and arrange a layer. Coarsely crumble over the feta cheese Silan and drizzle tablespoon olive oil and generously.

5. Serve immediately

Homemade Oven-Bake Tortilla Chips

Here's what you need:

- 12 gluten-free white corn tortillas
- Cooking spray
- ¼ teaspoon salt

Directions:

1. Place a rack in the middle of the oven. Preheat the oven to 375 ° F.

2. Line a 13 × 9-inch baking sheet (not nonstick) with foil.

3. Cut tortillas into wedges and place in single layer on prepared sheet. Spray lightly with cooking spray. Turn wedges over and spray other side. Lay an ovenproof wire rack on top to prevent the chips from curling. For curled chips choice, don't use the wire rack.

4. Bake the chips until they are crisp. Baking time will depend on the type and thickness of the tortillas you choose. Sprinkle the tortillas with salt as soon as you remove the chips from the oven and serve immediately.

Light and Tasty Fish Tacos

Here's what you need:

- 1 pound firm white fish (red snapper or tilapia)
- 3 tablespoons extra-virgin olive oil, divided
- 1 tablespoon fajita seasoning
- 1 small onion, thinly sliced
- 2 cups very thinly sliced green cabbage
- ½ cup chopped fresh cilantro
- ¼ cup plain yogurt or mayonnaise
- 2 tablespoons fresh lime juice
- 2 tablespoons rice vinegar
- 1 tablespoon sugar
- 1 teaspoon hot sauce
- ½ teaspoon salt
- ¼ teaspoons freshly ground black pepper
- 16 gluten-free corn tortillas (6-inch)
- 1 cup Monterey Jack cheese
- 1 cup homemade Pico de Gallo
- 1 ripe avocado, pitted and cut in 16 slices
- 1 can (11 ounces) mandarin oranges, drained
- 2 limes cut in halfS

Directions:

1. Brush the fish of your choice with 1 tablespoon oil and sprinkle with seasoning, pressing the seasoning into fish with fingers. Let the flavor sit for 15 minutes while the grill is heating.

2. Cook the onion in 1 tablespoon olive oil until very browned and soft, about 7 to 10 minutes. Transfer to a plate; cover with foil.

3. Cook the seasoned fish on grill until just done, for 8 to 10 minutes, depending on the cut (thickness) of the fish or until the crumbs are golden brown and the fish is just barely opaque when cut in the thickest part. Transfer to a serving plate and cover with foil to keep the temperature warm.

4. In a medium bowl, toss the cabbage with the remaining tablespoon of olive oil, and the cilantro, yogurt, lime juice, vinegar, sugar, hot sauce, salt, and pepper.

5. To assemble the tacos, soften the corn tortillas by wrapping a stack of them in wet paper towels or tea towels and steam them in a microwave on low for 5 minutes.

6. Place two tortillas together and fold them slightly in half. Fill each with 1/8 of the cheese, 1/8 of the onion, 1/8 of the fish, 1/8 of the cabbage, and 1/8 of the Pico de Gallo.

7. Top with slices of avocado and mandarin oranges.

8. Serve immediately with a squeeze of fresh lemon and enjoy!

Sweetly Treats and Smoothies for the Brain

Walnutty Fudge

Here's what you need:

- 8 oz. coconut oil
- 57 g almond butter, organic
- 34 g raw cacao, unsweetened
- 32 g walnuts, chopped
- 3 oz. maple syrup, organic
- 1 tsp. vanilla bean extract

Directions:

1. Place all of the above ingredients in a bowl and mix thoroughly.

2. Spread the mixture uniformly in a 5 x 9 sized glass baking dish.

3. Stick the baking dish in the freezer and leave it there for 30 minutes or more.

4. Reminder: Always keep the fudge on the fridge when not serving.

Chocolaty Cookie

Here's what you need:

- 8 oz. avocado slices, ripe
- 1 egg. organic
- 1 large banana, sliced
- 68 g raw cocoa, unsweetened
- ½ tsp. baking soda
- 1 tbsp. raw wild honey
- Semisweet chocolate chips (optional)

Directions:

1. First, heat up the oven to 350 F. In a mixing bowl, place the avocado slices and the banana slices.

2. Mash them together. Then, pour in the raw wild honey and mix well. Transfer the batter into a food processor.

3. Break in the egg. Add the cocoa and the baking powder. Pulse until completely blended.

4. Prepare a baking sheet by lining it with parchment paper. If you're using chocolate chips for this recipe, now is the time to stir them in.

5. Arrange spoonful of the dough on the baking dish while making sure that they're evenly spaced.

6. Place the baking dish in the oven and bake for about 9 minutes.

7. Serve and enjoy.

Super Easy and Sweet Parfaits

Here's what you need:

- 1 Gluten-free Double Chocolate Muffin (room temp)
- 1 cup vanilla yogurt
- 8 strawberries (stems removed, cut into slices)

Directions:

1. Simply cut the muffin into small cubes using a sharp knife.

2. After that, layer the vanilla yogurt, chocolate muffin cubes and fresh strawberries in a bowl.

3. Serve and enjoy.

Blueberry Ice Cream with Herbs

Here's what you need:

- 8 oz. blueberries
- 1 tsp. fresh rosemary, finely chopped
- 2 yolks from organic eggs
- 14 oz. coconut milk
- 2 tbsp. raw wild honey
- a teaspoonful of lemon juice

Directions:

1. In a food processor, mix the coconut milk and the blueberries. Add the honey and the lemon juice. Then also throw in the rosemary. Process until all the ingredients is completely blended.

2. Transfer the mixture into a pot. Adjust the stove's setting to medium heat. Add the egg yolks into the mixture. Bring the mixture to a low boil with continuous and brisk stirring.

3. As the mixture starts to boil, switch off the stove and leave it to cool at room temperature. Afterwards, pour the mixture into a bowl. Cover the bowl with cling wrap.

4. Place the bowl in the fridge and leave overnight. The following day, introduce the blend into an ice cream maker.

5. Then, spoon the ice cream into serving bowls.

Papaya and Apple Fusion

Here's what you need:

- 8 oz. papaya
- a couple of cupsful of baby spinach
- 1 medium-sized apple, core removed
- 6 oz. almond milk, unsweetened

Directions:

1. Combine all of the ingredients in a blender. Process until smooth. Enjoy your sweet and healthy treat!

Banana and Coconut Cookies

Here's what you need:

- 1 ripe banana, mashed
- 1 cup packed shredded coconut
- ¾ cup certified gluten-free oat flour or almond flour

Directions:

2. Start by preheating the oven to 350°, and line a baking sheet with parchment paper.

3. Next, mix the ingredients in a bowl and scoop batter into 1/8 measuring cup.

4. After that, invert and tap to empty the cookie batter onto the baking sheet from the first step.

5. Bake for 15 minutes or until both the outer edges and bottom of the cookies are browned.

6. Once that is achieved, you can take it out and serve with a dollop of peanut butter, seed butter, nut butter or jam if you want.

7. Serve and enjoy.

Frozen Strawberries and Avocado Smoothies

Here's what you need:

- ¼ cup coconut milk
- ¼ cup water
- 1 Tbsp raw unsalted sunflower seed kernels or almonds
- 1 Tbsp organic no sugar added sunflower seed butter or almond butter
- ¼ cup frozen strawberries, sliced
- ¼ ripe avocado, peeled and pit removed
- 1 Tbsp hemp hearts (hulled hemp seeds)
- ½ -inch piece of ginger root, peeled and chopped
- ½ tsp ground cinnamon

Directions:

1. Put all the ingredients together in a blender and blend until smooth. Serve and enjoy.

Blueberry and Avocado Smoothie

Here's what you need:

- A ripe banana
- 3-4 cubes of ice
- Ripe avocado
- Chia seeds
- Half cup of pomegranate juice

Directions:

1. Mix all the ingredients in a blender and blend until smooth. Serve and enjoy.

Boosting Avocado Smoothie

Here's what you need:

- ½ banana
- ½ cup blueberries
- 1 scoop vanilla whey protein powder
- ½ avocado
- 6 walnuts
- ½ cup water

Directions:

1. Just place all the ingredients together in a blender and blend until smooth and serve.

Blueberry Peach Smoothie

Here's what you need:

- 6 oz. blueberries
- 5 oz. water
- a couple of medium-sized peaches, pits removed
- a couple of leaves of collard greens
- 1 celery stalk

Directions:

1. Put all the ingredients together in a blender and blend until smooth. Serve and enjoy.

Pineapple and Kale Smoothie

Here's what you need:

- 4 oz. pineapple chunks
- 6 oz. water
- a couple of cupsful of kale, stem removed and leaves chopped to small pieces
- 1 medium-sized apple, core removed
- 1 medium-sized pear, core-removed

Directions:

1. Combine all the ingredients in a blender and blend until smooth. Serve and enjoy.

Peach Banana Smoothie

Here's what you need:

- 12 oz. apple juice, organic
- 2 tsp. raw wild honey
- ¾ cup peaches, ripe
- ¾ banana, sliced (without the peeling)
- 2 tsp. flaxseed oil
- 1 tbsp. vanilla-flavored yogurt
- 6 pcs. ice cubes

Directions:

1. Mix all the ingredients in a blender and then blend until smooth. Serve and enjoy.

Banana Avocado with Yogurt Smoothie

Here's what you need:

- a large-sized avocado
- a big banana
- 4 oz. yogurt
- 2 tbsp. raw wild honey
- 6 pcs. ice cubes

Directions:

1. Mix all the ingredients in a blender and blend until smooth. Serve and enjoy.

About the Author

The Health Buff is a group of writers that aims to help people on what diet they want to achieve. They explore a lot of dishes from different parts of the world and share them by putting everything into a book. These writers specifically share the diets and food that just actually worked for them.

The Health Buff writers are all food and health enthusiasts, thus, coming up with the idea of sharing what they all love to do to inspire other people to look after their health. They all believed that the best investment that you can ever make is in your own HEALTH.